My Mediterranean Dash Diet Cookbook

A Handful of Quick, Delicious Recipes for Your Mediterranean Dash Diet Meals

Kathyrn Solano

© Copyright 2021 - All rights reserved.

By reading this document, the reader agrees that under no circumstances is the author responsible for any losses, direct or indirect, which are incurred as a result of the use of information contained within this document, including, but not limited to, — errors, omissions, or inaccuracies.

Table of contents

BREAKFAST & LUNCH

Cauliflower Fritters With Hummus

Servings: 4

Cooking Time: 15 Minutes

Ingredients:

2 (15 oz) cans chickpeas, divided

2 1/2 tbsp olive oil, divided, plus more for frying

1 cup onion, chopped, about 1/2 a small onion

2 tbsp garlic, minced

2 cups cauliflower, cut into small pieces, about 1/2 a large head

1/2 tsp salt

black pepper

Topping:

Hummus, of choice

Green onion, diced

Directions:

Preheat oven to 400°F.

Rinse and drain 1 can of the chickpeas, place them on a paper towel to dry off well.

Then place the chickpeas into a large bowl, removing the loose skins that come off, and toss with 1 tbsp of olive oil, spread the chickpeas onto a large pan (being careful not to over-crowd them) and sprinkle with salt and pepper.

Bake for 20 minutes, then stir, and then bake an additional 5-10 minutes until very crispy

Once the chickpeas are roasted, transfer them to a large food processor and process until broken down and crumble - Don't over process them and turn it into flour, as you need to have some texture. Place the mixture into a small bowl, set aside.

In a large pan over medium-high heat, add the remaining 1 1/2 tbsp of olive oil.

Once heated, add in the onion and garlic, cook until lightly golden brown, about 2 minutes. Then add in the chopped cauliflower, cook for an additional 2 minutes, until the cauliflower is golden.

Turn the heat down to low and cover the pan, cook until the cauliflower is fork tender and the onions are golden brown and caramelized, stirring often, about 3-5 minutes.

Transfer the cauliflower mixture to the food processor, drain and rinse the remaining can of chickpeas and add them into the food processor, along with the salt and a pinch of pepper. Blend until smooth, and the mixture starts to ball, stop to scrape down the sides as needed.

Transfer the cauliflower mixture into a large bowl and add in 1/2 cup of the roasted chickpea crumbs (you won't use all of the crumbs, but it is easier to break them down when you have a larger amount.), stir until well combined.

In a large bowl over medium heat, add in enough oil to lightly cover the bottom of a large pan.

Working in batches, cook the patties until golden brown, about 2-3 minutes, flip and cook again.

Distribute among the container, placing parchment paper in between the fritters. Store in the fridge for 2-3 days.

To Serve: Heat through in the oven at 350F for 5-8 minutes. Top with hummus, green onion and enjoy!

Recipe Notes: Don't add too much oil while frying the fritter or they will end up soggy. Use only enough to cover the pan. Use a fork while frying and resist the urge to flip them every minute to see if they are golden.

Nutrition Info: Calories:333;Total Carbohydrates: 45g;
Total Fat: 13g;Protein: 14g

Italian Breakfast Sausage With Baby Potatoes And Vegetables

Servings: 4

Cooking Time: 30 Minutes

Ingredients:

1 lbs sweet Italian sausage links, sliced on the bias (diagonal)

2 cups baby potatoes, halved

2 cups broccoli florets

1 cup onions cut to 1-inch chunks

2 cups small mushrooms -half or quarter the large ones for uniform size

1 cup baby carrots

2 tbsp olive oil

1/2 tsp garlic powder

1/2 tsp Italian seasoning

1 tsp salt

1/2 tsp pepper

Directions:

Preheat the oven to 400 degrees F .

In a large bowl, add the baby potatoes, broccoli florets, onions, small mushrooms, and baby carrots.

Add in the olive oil, salt, pepper, garlic powder and Italian seasoning and toss to evenly coat.

Spread the vegetables onto a sheet pan in one even layer.

Arrange the sausage slices on the pan over the vegetables.

Bake for 30 minutes – make sure to sake halfway through to prevent sticking.

Allow to cool.

Distribute the Italian sausages and vegetables among the containers and store in the fridge for 2-3 days.

To Serve: Reheat in the microwave for 1-2 minutes, or until heated through and enjoy!

Recipe Notes: If you would like crispier potatoes, place them on the pan and bake for 15 minutes before adding the other ingredients to the pan.

Nutrition Info: Calories:321;Total Fat: 16g;Total Carbs: 23g;Fiber: 4g;Protein: 22g .

Greek Quinoa Breakfast Bowl

Servings: 6

Cooking Time: 20 Minutes

Ingredients:

12 eggs

¼ cup plain Greek yogurt

1 tsp onion powder

1 tsp granulated garlic

½ tsp salt

½ tsp pepper

1 tsp olive oil

1 (5 oz) bag baby spinach

1 pint cherry tomatoes, halved

1 cup feta cheese

2 cups cooked quinoa

Directions:

In a large bowl whisk together eggs, Greek yogurt, onion powder, granulated garlic, salt, and pepper, set aside

In a large skillet, heat olive oil and add spinach, cook the spinach until it is slightly wilted, about 3-4 minutes

Add in cherry tomatoes, cook until tomatoes are softened, 4 minutes

Stir in egg mixture and cook until the eggs are set, about 7-9 minutes, stir in the eggs as they cook to scramble

Once the eggs have set stir in the feta and quinoa, cook until heated through

Distribute evenly among the containers, store for 2-3 days

To serve: Reheat in the microwave for 30 seconds to 1 minute or heated through.

Nutrition Info: Calories:357; Total Carbohydrates: ; Total Fat: 20g.

Healthy Zucchini Kale Tomato Salad

Servings: 4

Cooking Time: 20 Minutes

Ingredients:

1 lb kale, chopped

2 tbsp fresh parsley, chopped

1 tbsp vinegar

1/2 cup can tomato, crushed

1 tsp paprika

1 cup zucchini, cut into cubes

1 cup grape tomatoes, halved

2 tbsp olive oil

1 onion, chopped

1 leek, sliced

Pepper

Salt

Directions:

Add oil into the inner pot of instant pot and set the pot on sauté mode.

Add leek and onion and sauté for 5 minutes.

Add kale and remaining ingredients and stir well.

Seal pot with lid and cook on high for 15 minutes.

Once done, allow to release pressure naturally for 10 minutes then release remaining using quick release. Remove lid.

Stir and serve.

Nutrition Info: Calories: 162; Fat: 3 g; Carbohydrates: 22.2 g; Sugar: 4.8 g; Protein: 5.2 g; Cholesterol: 0 mg .

Cheese And Cauliflower Frittata With Peppers

Servings: 6

Cooking Time: 30 Minutes

Ingredients:

10 eggs

1 seeded and chopped bell pepper

½ cup grated Parmigiano-Reggiano

½ cup milk, skim

½ teaspoon cayenne pepper

1 pound cauliflower, floret

½ teaspoon saffron

2 tablespoons chopped chives

Salt and black pepper as desired

Directions:

Prepare your oven by setting the temperature to 370 degrees Fahrenheit. You should also grease a skillet suitable for the oven.

In a medium-sized bowl, add the milk and eggs. Whisk them until they are frothy.

Sprinkle the grated Parmigiano-Reggiano cheese into the frothy mixture and fold the ingredients together.

Pour in the salt, saffron, cayenne pepper, and black pepper and gently stir.

Add in the chopped bell pepper and gently stir until the ingredients are fully incorporated.

Pour the egg mixture into the skillet and cook on medium heat over your stovetop for 4 minutes.

Steam the cauliflower florets in a pan. To do this, add ½ inch of water and ½ teaspoon sea salt. Pour in the cauliflower and cover for 3 to 8 minutes. Drain any extra water.

Add the cauliflower into the mixture and gently stir.

Set the skillet into the preheated oven and turn your timer to 13 minutes. Once the mixture is golden brown in the middle, remove the frittata from the oven.

Set your skillet aside for a couple of minutes so it can cool.

Slice and garnish with chives before you serve.

Nutrition Info: calories: 207, fats: grams, carbohydrates: 8 grams, protein: 17 grams.

Avocado Kale Omelette

Servings: 1

Cooking Time: 5 Minutes

Ingredients:

2 eggs

1 teaspoon milk

2 teaspoons olive oil

1 cup kale (chopped)

1 tablespoon lime juice

1 tablespoon cilantro (chopped)

1 teaspoon sunflower seeds

Pinch of red pepper (crushed)

¼ avocado (sliced)

sea salt or plain salt

freshly ground black pepper

Directions:

Toss all the Ingredients: (except eggs and milk) to make the kale

salad.

Beat the eggs and milk in a bowl.

Heat oil in a pan over medium heat. Then pour in the egg mixture and cook it until the bottom settles. Cook for 2 minutes and then flip it over and further cook for 20 seconds.

Finally, put the omelet in containers.

Top the omelet with the kale salad.

Serve warm.

Nutrition Info: Calories: 399, Total Fat: 28.8g, Saturated Fat: 6.2, Cholesterol: 328 mg, Sodium: 162 mg, Total Carbohydrate: 25.2g, Dietary Fiber: 6.3 g, Total Sugars: 9 g, Protein: 15.8 g, Vitamin D: 31 mcg, Calcium: 166 mg, Iron: 4 mg, Potassium: 980 mg

Mediterranean Breakfast Burrito

Servings: 6

Cooking Time: 5 Minutes

Ingredients:

9 eggs whole

6 tortillas whole 10 inch, regular or sun-dried tomato

3 tbsp sun-dried tomatoes, chopped

1/2 cup feta cheese I use light/low-fat feta

2 cups baby spinach washed and dried

3 tbsp black olives, sliced

3/4 cup refried beans, canned

Garnish:

Salsa

Directions:

Spray a medium frying pan with non- stick spray, add the eggs and scramble and toss for about 5 minutes, or until eggs are no longer liquid

Add in the spinach, black olives, sun-dried tomatoes and continue to stir and toss until no longer wet

Add in the feta cheese and cover, cook until cheese is melted

Add 2 tbsp of refried beans to each tortilla

Top with egg mixture, dividing evenly between all burritos, and wrap

Frying in a pan until lightly browned

Allow to cool completely before slicing

Wrap the slices in plastic wrap and then aluminum foil and place in the freezer for up to 2 months or fridge for 2 days

To Serve: Remove the aluminum foil and plastic wrap, and microwave for 2 minutes, then allow to rest for 30 seconds, enjoy! Enjoy hot with salsa and fruit

Nutrition Info: Calories:252; Total Carbohydrates: 21g;Total Fat: 11g;Protein: 14g |

Shakshuka With Feta

Servings: 4-6

Cooking Time:40 Minutes

Ingredients:

6 large eggs

3 tbsp extra-virgin olive oil

1 large onion, halved and thinly sliced

1 large red bell pepper, seeded and thinly sliced

3 garlic cloves, thinly sliced

1 tsp ground cumin

1 tsp sweet paprika

⅛ tsp cayenne, or to taste

1 (28-ounce) can whole plum tomatoes with juices, coarsely

chopped

¾ tsp salt, more as needed

¼ tsp black pepper, more as needed

5 oz feta cheese, crumbled, about 1 1/4 cups

To Serve:

Chopped cilantro

Hot sauce

Directions:

Preheat oven to 375 degrees F

In a large skillet over medium-low heat, add the oil

Once heated, add the onion and bell pepper, cook gently until very soft, about 20 minutes

Add in the garlic and cook until tender, 1 to 2 minutes, then stir in cumin, paprika and cayenne, and cook 1 minute

Pour in tomatoes, season with 3/4 tsp salt and 1/4 tsp pepper, simmer until tomatoes have thickened, about 10 minutes

Then stir in crumbled feta

Gently crack eggs into skillet over tomatoes, season with salt and pepper

Transfer skillet to oven

Bake until eggs have just set, 7 to 10 minutes

Allow to cool and distribute among the containers, store in the fridge for 2-3 days

To Serve: Reheat in the oven at 360 degrees F for 5 minutes or until heated through

Nutrition Info: Calories:337; Carbs: 17g; Total Fat: 25g;Protein.

Spinach, Feta And Egg Breakfast Quesadillas

Servings: 5

Cooking Time: 15 Minutes

Ingredients:

8 eggs (optional)

2 tsp olive oil

1 red bell pepper

1/2 red onion

1/4 cup milk

4 handfuls of spinach leaves

1 1/2 cup mozzarella cheese

5 sun-dried tomato tortillas

1/2 cup feta

1/4 tsp salt

1/4 tsp pepper

Spray oil

Directions:

In a large non-stick pan over medium heat, add the olive oil.

Once heated, add the bell pepper and onion, cook for 4-5 minutes until soft

In the meantime, whisk together the eggs, milk, salt and pepper in a bowl.

Add in the egg/milk mixture into the pan with peppers and onions, stirring

frequently, until eggs are almost cooked through.

Add in the spinach and feta, fold into the eggs, stirring until spinach is wilted and eggs are cooked through.

Remove the eggs from heat and plate

Spray a separate large non-stick pan with spray oil, and place over medium heat.

Add the tortilla, on one half of the tortilla, spread about ½ cup of the egg mixture.

Top the eggs with around ⅓ cup of shredded mozzarella cheese.

Fold the second half of the tortilla over, then cook for 2 minutes, or until golden brown.

Flip and cook for another minute until golden brown.

Allow the quesadilla to cool completely, divide among the container, store for 2 days or wrap in plastic wrap and foil, and freeze for up to 2 months.

To Serve: Reheat in oven at 375 for 3-5 minutes or until heated through.

25

Nutrition Info: (1/2 quesadilla): Calories:213;Total Fat: 11g;Total Carbs: 15g;Protein: 15g

Breakfast Cobbler

Servings: 4

Cooking Time: 12 Minutes

Ingredients:

2 lbs apples, cut into chunks

1 1/2 cups water

1/4 tsp nutmeg

1 1/2 tsp cinnamon

1/2 cup dry buckwheat

1/2 cup dates, chopped

Pinch of ground ginger

Directions:

Spray instant pot from inside with cooking spray.

Add all ingredients into the instant pot and stir well.

Seal pot with a lid and select manual and set timer for 12 minutes.

Once done, release pressure using quick release. Remove lid.

Stir and serve.

Nutrition Info: Calories: 195; Fat: 0.9 g; Carbohydrates: 48.3 g; Sugar: 25.8 g; Protein: 3.3 g; Cholesterol: 0 mg

Egg-topped Quinoa Bowl With Kale

Servings: 2

Cooking Time: 5 Minutes

Ingredients:

1-ounce pancetta, chopped

1 bunch kale, sliced

½ cup cherry tomatoes, halved

1 teaspoon red wine vinegar

1 cup cooked quinoa

1 teaspoon olive oil

2 eggs

1/3 cup avocado, sliced

sea salt or plain salt

fresh black pepper

Directions:

Start by heating pancetta in a skillet until golden brown. Add in kale and further cook for 2 minutes.

Then, stir in tomatoes, vinegar, and salt and remove from heat.

Now, divide this mixture into 2 bowls, add avocado to both, and then set aside.

Finally, cook both the eggs and top each bowl with an egg.

Serve hot with toppings of your choice.

Nutrition Info: Calories: 547, Total Fat: 22., Saturated Fat: 5.3, Cholesterol: 179 mg, Sodium: 412 mg, Total Carbohydrate: 62.5 g, Dietary Fiber: 8.6 g, Total Sugars: 1.7 g, Protein: 24.7 g, Vitamin D: 15 mcg, Calcium: 117 mg, Iron: 6 mg, Potassium: 1009 mg

Strawberry Greek Frozen Yogurt

Servings: 5

Cooking Time: 2-4 Hours

Ingredients:

3 cups plain Greek low-fat yogurt

1 cup sugar

¼ cup lemon juice, freshly squeezed

2 teaspoons vanilla

1/8 teaspoon salt

1 cup strawberries, sliced

Directions:

In a medium-sized bowl, add yogurt, lemon juice, sugar, vanilla, and salt.

Whisk the whole mixture well.

Freeze the yogurt mix in a 2-quart ice cream maker according to the given instructions.

During the final minute, add the sliced strawberries.

Transfer the yogurt to an airtight container.

Place in the freezer for 2-4 hours.

Remove from the freezer and allow it to stand for 5-15 minutes. Serve and enjoy!

30

Nutrition Info: 251, Total Fat: 0.5 g, Saturated Fat: 0.1 g, Cholesterol: 3 mg, Sodium: 130 mg, Total Carbohydrate: 48.7 g, Dietary Fiber: 0.6 g, Total Sugars: 47.3 g, Protein: 14.7 g, Vitamin D: 1 mcg, Calcium: 426 mg, Iron: 0 mg, Potassium: 62 mg

Peanut Butter Banana Pudding

Servings: 1

Cooking Time: 25 Minutes

Ingredients:

2 bananas, halved

¼ cup smooth peanut butter

Coconut for garnish, shredded

Directions:

Start by blending bananas and peanut butter in a blender and mix until smooth or desired texture obtained.

Pour into a bowl and garnish with coconut if desired.

Enjoy.

Nutrition Info: Calories: 589, Total Fat: 33.3g, Saturated Fat: 6.9, Cholesterol: 0 mg, Sodium: 13 mg, Total Carbohydrate: 66.5 g, Dietary Fiber: 10 g, Total Sugars: 38 g, Protein: 18.8 g, Vitamin D: 0 mcg, Calcium: 40 mg, Iron: 2 mg, Potassium: 1264 mg

Almond Peach Oatmeal

Servings: 2

Cooking Time: 10 Minutes

Ingredients:

1 cup unsweetened almond milk

2 cups of water

1 cup oats

2 peaches, diced

Pinch of salt

Directions:

Spray instant pot from inside with cooking spray.

Add all ingredients into the instant pot and stir well.

Seal pot with a lid and select manual and set timer for 10 minutes.

Once done, allow to release pressure naturally for 10 minutes then release remaining using quick release. Remove lid.

Stir and serve.

Nutrition Info: Calories: 234; Fat: 4.8 g; Carbohydrates: 42.7 g; Sugar: 9 g; Protein: 7.3 g; Cholesterol: 0 mg

Coconut And Banana Mix

Servings: 4

Cooking Time: 4 Minutes

Ingredients:

1 cup coconut milk

1 banana

1 cup dried coconut

2 tablespoons ground flax seed

3 tablespoons chopped raisins

⅛ teaspoon nutmeg

⅛ teaspoon cinnamon

Salt to taste

Directions:

Set a large skillet on the stove and set it to low heat.

Chop up the banana.

Pour the coconut milk, nutmeg, and cinnamon into the skillet.

Pour in the ground flaxseed while stirring continuously.

Add the dried coconut and banana. Mix the ingredients until combined well.

Allow the mixture to simmer for 2 to 3 minutes while stirring occasionally.

Set four airtight containers on the counter.

Remove the pan from heat and sprinkle enough salt for your taste buds.

Divide the mixture into the containers and place them into the fridge overnight. They can remain in the fridge for up to 3 days.

Before you set this tasty mixture in the microwave to heat up, you need to let it thaw on the counter for a bit.

Nutrition Info: calories: 279, fats: 22 grams, carbohydrates: 25 grams, protein: 6.4 grams.

Raspberry-lemon Olive Oil Muffins

Servings: 12

Cooking Time: 20 Minutes

Ingredients:

Cooking spray to grease baking liners

1 cup all-purpose flour

1 cup whole-wheat flour

½ cup tightly packed light brown sugar

½ teaspoon baking soda

½ teaspoon aluminum-free baking powder

⅛ teaspoon kosher salt

1¼ cups buttermilk

1 large egg

¼ cup extra-virgin olive oil

1 tablespoon freshly squeezed lemon juice

Zest of 2 lemons

1¼ cups frozen raspberries (do not thaw)

Directions:

Preheat the oven to 400°F and line a muffin tin with baking liners. Spray the liners lightly with cooking spray.

In a large mixing bowl, whisk together the all-purpose flour, whole-wheat flour, brown sugar, baking soda, baking powder, and salt.

In a medium bowl, whisk together the buttermilk, egg, oil, lemon juice, and lemon zest.

Pour the wet ingredients into the dry ingredients and stir just until blended. Do not overmix.

Fold in the frozen raspberries.

Scoop about ¼ cup of batter into each muffin liner and bake for 20 minutes, or until the tops look browned and a paring knife comes out clean when inserted. Remove the muffins from the tin to cool.

STORAGE: Store covered containers at room temperature for up to 4 days. To freeze muffins for up to 3 months, wrap them in foil and place in an airtight resealable bag.

Nutrition Info: Total calories: 166; Total fat: 5g; Saturated fat: 1g; Sodium: 134mg; Carbohydrates: 30g; Fiber: 3g; Protein: 4g

Mushroom Tomato Egg Cups

Servings: 4

Cooking Time: 5 Minutes

Ingredients:

4 eggs

1/2 cup tomatoes, chopped

1/2 cup mushrooms, chopped

2 tbsp fresh parsley, chopped

1/4 cup half and half

1/2 cup cheddar cheese, shredded

Pepper

Salt

Directions:

In a bowl, whisk the egg with half and half, pepper, and salt.

Add tomato, mushrooms, parsley, and cheese and stir well.

Pour egg mixture into the four small jars and seal jars with lid.

Pour 1 1/2 cups of water into the instant pot then place steamer rack in the pot.

Place jars on top of the steamer rack.

Seal pot with lid and cook on high for 5 minutes.

Once done, release pressure using quick release. Remove lid.

Serve and enjoy.

Nutrition Info: Calories: 146;Fat: 10.g;Carbohydrates: 2.5 g;Sugar: 1.2 g;Protein: 10 g;Cholesterol: 184 mg.

GREAT MEDITERRANEAN DIET RECIPES

Tabbouleh

Preparation time: 30 minutes

Cooking time: 0 minute

Servings: 4

Ingredients:

One cup bulgur

One cup sliced Cucumbers

One cup sliced Radish

Four sliced scallions

One bunch of Chopped mint leaves

2 tbsp lemon juice

½ cup olive oil

Pepper to taste

Kosher salt to taste

Directions :

Fill a large bowl halfway with hot tap water and stir bulgur into it for 20 to 30 minutes. Let it absorb water enough to not be mushy but soft. In a large bowl, put mint and the vegetables sliced earlier. Drain excess water off the bulgur by squeezing, one at a time. Squeeze tightly by holding it over a sink or a sieve, adding each bulgur squeezed into the vegetable bowl.

Add olive oil and lemon juice into the salad. Blend all the ingredients by using either a large spoon or hands. Add salt and pepper with seasoning to taste (if desired).

Serve it as a side dish for dinner or with crusty bread as a lunch. Enjoy!

Nutrition Info: Calories: 367 kcal Fat: 28 g Protein: 5 g Carbs: 29 g Fiber: 7 g

Stuffed Poblano Peppers

Preparation time: 20 minutes

Cooking time: 30 minutes

Servings: 5

Ingredients:

46 g Poblano peppers

Two cups of water

One cup quinoa

3 tbsp olive oil

One diced onion

Two diced ribs celery

Two diced carrots

Two minced garlic cloves

½ cup diced red peppers roasted

1 tbsp adobo sauce with chipotle

One cup peas

1/3 cup chopped pecans

Directions :

Heat the oven before 375°F. With stem, slit each pepper lengthwise. Scoop the seeds out and put them aside. Take a medium saucepan, heat water, and add quinoa. Until cooked, boil it and simmer with water immersed. Put it aside. Add olive oil in a medium heated skillet.

Sauté the carrots, onion, and celery for about 8 minutes until softened. Then add garlic and for a minute sauté it. Add quinoa cooked before in it and mix well. Add the chipotle, pecans, peas, and roasted red peppers. A shallow baking dish places stuffed peppers and bake them until the peppers are softened for 30 minutes. Serve with meat or a side salad. Enjoy!

Nutrition Info: Calories: 302 kcal Fat: 16 g Protein: 8 g Carbs: 34 g Fiber: 7 g

Shiitake, Soba Noodles, and Miso Bowl

Preparation time: 5 minutes

Cooking time: 15 minutes

Servings: 2

Ingredients:

Three cups of water

½ cup dried shiitake mushrooms

4 oz soba noodles

1 tbsp white miso

Directions :

In a medium saucepan, boil water over high heat. Add mushrooms and cook them for 6 minutes until swollen and softened. Add in the noodles and cook until al dente. Measure one by 4 cups of noodle broth. Add the miso to it and mix thoroughly with a fork or whisk.

Pour this mixture back into the saucepan. Serve in bowls. Enjoy!

Nutrition Info: Calories: 156 kcal Fat: 1 g Protein: 8 g Carbs: 33 g Fiber: 6 g

Collard and Rice Stuffed Red Peppers

Preparation time: 10 minutes

Cooking time: 50 minutes

Servings: 4

Ingredients:

Two red bell peppers

2 tbsp olive oil

Black pepper to taste

Six cups collard greens

½ chopped sweet onion

Three minced garlic cloves

One cup of white rice cooked

2 tbsp lemon Juice

¼ cup roasted sunflower seeds

Directions :

Preheat oven at 400°F.

Cut half the peppers and remove the stems and seeds. Brush the inside and out with one tbsp of olive oil. Spice them with pepper and put the baking dish cut side down.

Until just tender, bake them for ten to fifteen minutes. Flip-up the cut-side of peppers after removing them from the oven and leave the oven on.

Take a large saucepan and boil four cups of water. Cook collard greens in it until just tender, for about five to seven minutes. Drain and rinse them under cold water. Then Chop them finely. Take a large skillet, and at medium heat, put the left behind tbsp of olive oil. Add in the onion, stir and cook for five to seven minutes, until it turns brown. Add in and cook garlic until it is fragrant. Mix in the collard greens. Put it off from the stove, and add rice and lemon juice in it. Spice it up with pepper.

Divide this filling into the pepper halves and crest each half with one tbsp of sunflower seeds. Add one by the fourth cup of water in a baking dish, wrap it with aluminum foil. Bake it for twenty minutes, until it is heated through. Uncover it and then bake again for five more minutes.

Nutrition Info: Calories: 217 kcal Fat: 12 g Protein: 6 g Carbs: 24 g Fiber: 5 g

Winter Minestrone

Preparation time: 35 minutes

Cooking time: 60 minutes

Servings:6

Ingredients:

Two cups chopped cabbage

One cup chopped cauliflower florets

One cup chopped butternut squash

½ cup chopped onion

½ cup chopped carrot

½ cup diced celery

Eight cups water

½ black beans

5 oz small macaroni

¼ grated Parmesan cheese

¼ olive oil

Salt to taste

Black pepper to taste

Directions :

Mix all the vegetables chopped in a Dutch oven or large pot. Stir fry for two minutes.

Cover it up with water and set it above medium-high heat. Add in the macaroni, grated cheese, olive oil, and beans. Bring it to a boil. Lessen the heat to cook and simmer for one hour.

Add season as needed with pepper, salt, and extra cheese if preferred. The soup must be thick.

Present in bowls with a garnishing of grated cheese on top of it.

Nutrition Info: Calories: 249 kcal Fat: 11 g Protein: 4 g Carbs: 35 g Fiber: 5 g

Penne with Tomato, Basil and Parmesan Cheese

Preparation time: 5 minutes

Cooking time: 20 minutes

Servings: 4

Ingredients:

Twelve cups water

Three cups dry penne

3 tbsp olive oil extra virgin

12 oz grape tomatoes

2 tbsp minced garlic

One cup chopped basil

4 tbsp shredded parmesan cheese

Directions :

Boil a large pot of water. Add pasta and cook for twelve minutes, or until al dente. Occasionally stir it. Drain the cooked pasta using a strainer and put it aside. Add and heat two tbsp of olive oil to a medium-sized saucepan over medium-high heat. Once it is hot, add and sauté tomatoes until they are soft for almost two minutes. Put garlic and cook for an extra minute.

Add pasta and also leftover tbsp of olive oil to the saucepan, and fry for 1 min.

Add three by four cups of basil and toss the pan until it is evenly distributed.

Adorn it with leftover parmesan cheese and chopped basil, and serve right away.

Nutrition Info: Calories: 406 kcal Fat: 13 g Protein: 15 g Carbs: 69 g Fiber: 4 g

Delightful Bulgur Pilaf

Preparation time: 15 minutes

Cooking time: 10 minutes

Servings: 5

Ingredients:

One cup of water

One chopped tomato

One cup bulgur wheat

One cup corn kernels

¼ cup dill

Directions :

Take a tomato, bulgur, and water and boil it in a saucepan over high heat. Put in dill and corn and reduce the heat. Fry for almost five minutes frequently.

If required and one by the fourth cup, add more water until the bulgur is not soggy but tender.

Until the water is absorbed, Cook it. It turns into a pilaf, like rice cooked with other ingredients.

Remove from the stove. Wrap and let stand for five to seven minutes.

Serve with a green salad for lunch or as a side dish to seafood or meat for dinner. Enjoy!

Nutrition Info: Calories: 157 kcal Fat: 0.8 g Protein: 6 g Carbs: 35 g Fiber: 6 g

Corn Pudding

Preparation time: 10 minutes

Cooking time: 40 minutes

Servings: 6

Ingredients:

Butter

2 tbsp all-purpose flour

½ tsp baking soda

Three eggs

¾ cup of rice milk

3 tbsp melted butter

2 tbsp light sour cream

2 tbsp granulated sugar

Two cups corn kernels

Directions :

Heat the oven before 350°F. Lightly lubricate with butter an eight by an eight-inch baking dish, and put it aside. Take a small bowl, mix flour and baking soda substitute, and put it aside.

Take a medium-sized bowl and beat together sugar, butter, sour cream, eggs, and rice milk.

Blend the egg mixture into the flour mixture until even. Mix the corn to the mixture and stir until even. Spoon this mixture in the baking dish and bake until the pudding is set, for almost forty minutes. Let it cool for fifteen minutes and serve warm.

Nutrition Info: Calories: 180 kcal Fat: 10 g Protein: 5 g Carbs: 21 g Fiber: 6 g

Egg White Frittata with Penne

Preparation time: 15 minutes

Cooking time: 30 minutes

Servings: 4-5

Ingredients:

Six egg whites

¼ cup of rice milk

1 tbsp chopped parsley

1 tbsp chopped thyme

1 tsp chopped chives

Black pepper to taste

2 tbsp olive oil

¼ chopped sweet onion

1 tsp minced garlic

½ cup chopped red bell pepper (boiled)

Two cups cooked penne

Directions :

Heat the oven at 350°F prior.

Whisk egg whites, chives, parsley, rice milk thyme, and pepper in a large bowl.

Warm olive oil over medium heat in an ovenproof frying pan. Fry the garlic, red pepper, and onion for four min until they are soft. Add the cooked penne to the frying pan using a spatula to pour the pasta evenly. Cover the pasta with egg mixture and shake the pan, distribute it evenly.

Set the frittata's bottom, leave the frying pan on the heat for one minute, and then move the pan to the oven. Bake it for twenty-five min until it is golden brown and set.

Take it out from the oven and dish it up immediately.

Nutrition Info: Calories: 173 kcal Fat: 3 g Protein: 10 g Carbs: 25 g Fiber: 2 g

Coconut and Kidney Bean

Preparation time: 15 minutes

Cooking time: 0 minute

Servings: 4

Ingredients:

2 tbsp olive oil

One diced onion

Two minced garlic cloves

1/3 diced green pepper

½ minced jalapeño pepper

6 oz kidney beans

One cup of coconut milk

Two cups white rice

¼ tsp black pepper

One chopped thyme sprig

½ tsp sea salt

Directions :

Heat at medium heat olive oil in a saucepan. Add garlic,

peppers, and onion. Reduce heat and fry for ten min until it turns soft. Add in coconut milk and kidney beans to the cooked veggies.

Add the cooked rice, pepper, and salt, if needed. Put a sprig of fresh thyme.

Cook and blend carefully, wrap it tightly, for ten to fifteen min on low heat. Enjoy!

Nutrition Info: Calories: 141 kcal Fat: 10 g Protein: 11 g Carbs: 1 g Fiber: 1.8 g

Venezuelan Corn Fritter (Arepas)

Preparation time: 20 minutes

Cooking time: 25 minutes

Servings: 12

Ingredients:

Two corn

Two sliced scallions

One sliced jalapeño

1/3 cup yellow cornmeal

½ cup flour

1 tsp sugar

¼ tsp salt

½ tsp baking soda

2 tbsp butter

One egg

½ cup whole milk

2.5 cup canola oil

One bunch of Papallo leaves

¼ cup sour cream

Directions :

Take a large pot; boil enough water to cover the corns.

Add corns and cook for five min until they are tender. Cool them, and then into a mixing bowl, slice off the kernels. Add flour, scallions, cornmeal, jalapeños, sugar, baking soda, and salt to the bowl. In a small saucepan, melt the butter, whisk the melted butter, milk, and egg together in another separate bowl. Pour this mixture into the dry ingredients and blend well. Over medium-high heat, add and Heat oil in a large skillet. Add a heaping tbsp of corn batter in oil and spread it to make a pancake of three and a half inches across.

Cook it until it is set on one side, then turn over and continue until it turns light brown. Two to three min on each side. Sap on paper towels. Repeat this process until all the batter is gone. Add extra oil, if needed. Dish out with a little crème Fraiche in the core of pancake, if needed, and dust with a cilantro leaf. Enjoy!

Nutrition Info: Calories: 284 kcal Fat: 18 g Protein: 6 g Carbs: 27 g Fiber: 1 g

Broccoli Cauliflower Carrot Bake

Preparation time: 5 minutes

Cooking time: 50 minutes

Servings: 12

Ingredients:

3 cups broccoli

One cup carrots

Two cups cauliflower

4 tbsp butter

2 tbsp flour

One pinch of pepper

One cup of milk

One cup chopped onions

3 oz softened cream cheese

½ cup shredded sharp cheddar cheese

½ cup soft bread crumbs

Directions :

Heat oven at 350 degrees prior. Wash and dice vegetables;
steam until they are crisp but tender, and drain them. Melt two

tbsp of butter in a saucepan. Mix pepper and flour, and then pour milk. Cook and whisk until thick and bubbly. Mix cream cheese until it is even on low heat.

Lay vegetables in half quarter casserole dish and put the sauce over, mix lightly.

Put shredded cheese over the top and Bake for about fifteen minutes.

Put bread crumbs and leftover butter and dust over on casserole. Bake for twenty-five more min.

Nutrition Info: Calories: 116 kcal Fat: 9 g Protein: 4 g Carbs: 7 g Fiber: 1 g

Roasted Fall Vegetables

Preparation time: 20 minutes

Cooking time: 30 minutes

Servings: 8

Ingredients:

One sliced potato

One sliced sweet potato

Four sliced and peeled shallots

One sliced acorn squash

Two sliced parsnips

Two sliced turnips

¼ olive oil

Black pepper

6 tbsp butter

Four sage leaves

2 tsp Spanish sherry vinegar

One pinch of sea salt

Directions :

Heat oven to 400°F prior. Take a large bowl and put vegetables in it.

Mix olive oil and season with pepper and salt, if needed. Flip to mix well.

Lay vegetables on a baking sheet lined with dish or parchment. Cook, or until vegetables are roasted to sweetness or browned for thirty min. Over medium heat, melt butter in a small saucepan or frying pan. Tear up sage leaves and put them in the saucepan.

Remove from heat when the butter gets brown but does not burn. Mix vinegar, salt, and pepper according to taste. Lay each portion of vegetables on its plate. Sprinkle enough of the sage butter to enhance their taste, but don't soak. Enjoy!

Nutrition Info: Calories: 211 kcal Fat: 16 g Protein: 2 g Carbs: 18 g Fiber: 3 g

Chickpea Turnip Greens Tacos

Preparation time: 10 minutes

Cooking time: 0 minute

Servings: 12

Ingredients:

6 oz chickpeas

One minced red onion

One minced garlic

Black pepper

1 tbsp lemon juice

1 tbsp chopped parsley

½ tbsp olive oil

10 oz turnip greens

12 corn tortillas

One shredded cucumber

2 oz crumbled Feta cheese

¼ tsp sea salt

Directions :

Mix garlic, onions, and chickpeas in a large bowl. Spice with salt and pepper, according to taste.

Add olive oil, parsley, and lemon juice. Mix until it turns into a chunky paste. Put in thawed turnip greens into this mixture. Mix. Take a warmed corn tortilla (in a skillet or the oven, if you prefer) and put some chickpea turnip greens batter. Dish out with feta cheese and shredded cucumber garnish. Enjoy!

Nutrition Info: Calories: 257 kcal Fat: 8 g Protein: 9 g Carbs: 39 g Fiber: 8 g

Soy Ginger Roasted Eggplant

Preparation time: 10 minutes

Cooking time: 40 minutes

Servings: 4

Ingredients:

Two eggplants

2 tbsp low sodium soy sauce

½ tsp garlic powder

1 tsp ground ginger

2 tsp olive oil

1/8 tsp pepper

Directions :

Heat oven at 400°F prior. Cut the bottom and stem end from the eggplants. Then slice in half each eggplant lengthwise. Cut deep diagonal lines deep into the eggplant's flesh about one inch apart, but avoid slicing through the skin. Turn it over and do the same to make a diamond-shaped pattern. Take a small bowl and add olive oil, pepper, soy sauce, ground ginger, and garlic powder. Evenly wrap the eggplant's flesh side of each half with soy sauce mixture. Lay the halves' flesh side down onto a foil-lined baking sheet or parchment. Roast in the oven for thirty to forty min, until the flesh side is browned and caramelized and the skin look collapsed.

Once they are cooked through and soft, take it out from the oven, flip the side with the skin side down to cool. Enjoy at room temperature or warm.

Nutrition Info: Calories: 144 kcal Fat: 7 g Protein: 3 g Carbs: 20 g Fiber: 5 g

Vegan Shortbread Cookies

Preparation time: 5 minutes

Cooking time: 20 minutes

Servings: 8

Ingredients:

¼ cup of coconut oil

½ cup Powdered sugar

2.5 tbsp yogurt

1 tsp Vanilla extract

½ tsp Cardamom

¼ tsp Salt

1/8 tsp Baking soda

½ cup Whole wheat flour

One cup flour

1/8 cup chopped cranberries

1/8 cup chopped Apricots

1/8 cup chopped Pecans

Directions :

Preheat the oven to 325 degrees. Cream the sugar, coconut oil, and non-dairy yogurt until they become creamy and smooth. Use the hand mixer. Add in the cardamom and vanilla; Mix (for 30-45 seconds). In the flour, now add the salt and baking soda. Mix well using a mixing spoon the ½ cup of the flour mixture in the coconut oil mixture.

Do not add flour more than ½ cup at a time to form a soft, fluffy dough. If the mixture becomes too dry, add a tsp. of water. If the mixture becomes too sticky, add a tbsp of flour.

Add the nuts and dried fruit to the mixture for this step. Work it thoroughly.

Take a 1 to 1 ½ -inch wide log and shape the prepared dough into it. Take a parchment sheet and fold it over the log. Now, freeze for about thirty minutes. Take the log out from the freezer and slice it into ¼ inch slices (or as desired). Take a parchment-lined baking sheet and place the dough on it. For 18-20 minutes, bake it. Adjust the temperature of your oven for the best results. Cool and store! (in an airtight container)

Nutrition Info: Calories: 203 kcal Fat: 9 g Protein: 3 g Carbs: 29 g Fiber: 2 g

Glazed Green Beans

Preparation time: 5 minutes

Cooking time: 15 minutes

Servings: 6

Ingredients:

12 cups Water

1.5 lb green beans

1 tbsp olive oil

½ tbsp lemon juice

Black pepper to taste Sauce

1 tsp Canola oil

1 tbsp Honey

One minced garlic clove

1 tsp Water

Directions :

Take a stock-pot. Add water to it and bring it to a boil. Add beans to the water, and cook them until they start turning bright green (for 3 minutes). Be careful not to overcook. Take the beans; rinse and drain with cold water (for about 1 minute).

Place them in a bowl and pat them dry thoroughly. Now, set aside. Take separately honey, garlic, 1 tsp. Oil and water; Whisk to make a sauce. Now set aside. Heat one tbsp. Oil in a large pan (medium heat). Add beans to the pan, and stir the beans to coat with oil. Add sauce, continuing to stir, and cook for additional 3 minutes. Finished green beans will be bright green and crisp-tender.

Before serving, season the dish with freshly ground black pepper and lemon juice.

Nutrition Info: Calories: 70 kcal Fat: 3 g Protein: 2 g Carbs: 11 g Fiber: 4 g

Spicy roasted red pepper hummus

Preparation time: 15 minutes

Cooking time: 60 minutes

Servings: 8

Ingredients:

½ tsp cumin

15 oz garbanzo beans

1.5 tbsp tahini

4 oz roasted red pepper

One minced garlic clove

½ tsp cayenne pepper

3 tbsp lemon juice

¼ tsp salt

1 tbsp chopped parsley

Directions :

Blend all the ingredients in the blender and refrigerator for an hour before serving.

Nutrition Info: Calories: 64.2 kcal Fat: 2.2 g Protein: 2.5 g Carbs: 9.6 g Fiber: 2.1

Simple Mediterranean olive oil pasta

Preparation time: 10 minutes

Cooking time: 9 minutes

Servings: 5

Ingredients:

1 lb spaghetti

Four crushed garlic cloves,

½ cup Olive Oil

Salt to taste

12 oz halved grape tomatoes

1 cup chopped parsley

Red pepper flakes crushed

Three chopped scallions

6 oz marinated artichoke hearts

1 tsp black pepper

¼ cup halved pitted olives

12 torn basil leaves

¼ cup crumbled feta cheese

Zest of one lemon

Directions :

Cook pasta according to the instructions given on the box. Sauté garlic and salt in heated olive oil over medium flame. Add tomatoes, scallions, and parsley. Cook for one minute. Pour the garlic sauce over the cooked and drained pasta. Sprinkle pepper and leftover ingredients and toss well.

Nutrition Info: Calories: 389 kcal Fat: 16.6 g Protein: 10.7 g Carbs: 51.1 g Fiber: 11 g

Roasted vegetable barley

Preparation time: 10 minutes

Cooking time: 40 minutes

Servings: 6

Ingredients:

1 cup pearl barley

Two diced zucchini squash

water

One diced bell pepper (red and yellow)

2 oz chopped parsley

salt to taste

One diced red onion

black pepper to taste

¾ tsp smoked paprika

2 tsp harissa spice

Olive oil

One minced garlic clove

Two chopped scallions

Feta cheese

2 tbsp lemon juice

Toasted pine nuts

Directions :

Boil barley in water for 45 minutes. In a bowl, mix veggies, salt, harissa spice, paprika, pepper, and oil. Roast in a preheated oven at 425 degrees for 25 minutes. Transfer the roasted veggies, cooked barley, scallions, parsley, garlic, lemon juice, and oil in a large bowl and mix to coat well.

Nutrition Info: Calories: 192 kcal Fat: 5.4 g Protein: 4.6 g Carbs: 33.2 g Fiber: 2.1 g

Moroccan couscous

Preparation time: 10 minutes

Cooking time: 10 minutes

Servings: 5

Ingredients:

2 cups couscous

4 cups flavorful stock

2 tbsp olive oil

1 tsp salt

1/2 tsp black pepper

Directions :

Boil stock, oil, salt, and pepper in the pot.

Transfer the potting mixture to a bowl, add couscous and toss.

Nutrition Info: Calories: 226 kcal Fat: 5 g Protein: 7 g Carbs: 37 g Fiber: 2 g

Mushroom barley soup

Preparation time: 15 minutes

Cooking time: 60 minutes

Servings: 4

Ingredients:

Olive oil

16 oz sliced Bella mushrooms

Kosher salt to taste

One chopped yellow onion,

Four minced garlic cloves

Two chopped celery stalks

One diced carrot

8 oz chopped white mushrooms

½ cup crushed tomatoes

Black pepper to taste

1 tsp coriander

½ tsp smoked paprika

½ tsp cumin

6 cups broth

1 cup pearl barley

½ cup chopped parsley

Directions :

Cook mushrooms in heated olive oil over a high flame in a Dutch oven for seven minutes and keep it aside. Sauté onions, carrots, white mushrooms, and celery in the same pan with more olive oil for five minutes over medium flame. Sprinkle pepper and salt. Stir in tomatoes and spices. Cook for five more minutes. Mix barley and broth and boil for five minutes.
Simmer it for 45 minutes over low flame. Add cooked mushrooms and cook for few more minutes. Sprinkle parsley and serve.

Nutrition Info: Calories: 198 kcal Fat: 9.9 g Protein: 5.8 g Carbs: 24 g Fiber: 5.8 g

Mediterranean couscous salad

Preparation time: 15 minutes

Cooking time: 10 minutes

Servings: 6

Ingredients:

Lemon-Dill Vinaigrette

1 tbsp lemon juice

1/3 cup olive oil

1 tsp dill

1.5 minced garlic cloves

Salt to taste

Black pepper to taste

Israeli Couscous

2 cups Pearl Couscous

3 oz mozzarella cheese

Water

Olive oil

2 cups grape tomatoes

1/2 chopped English cucumber

1/3 cup chopped red onions

15 oz chickpeas

½ cup Kalamata olives

14 oz chopped artichoke hearts

18 chopped basil leaves

Directions :

Mix all the ingredients of vinaigrette in a container and set aside. The lemon dill vinaigrette is ready. Cook couscous in heated olive oil over medium flame. Pour boiling water about three cups and cook until couscous is cooked. Combine all the leftover ingredients in a bowl except mozzarella. Mix couscous with the ingredients. Pour vinaigrette and toss well. Sprinkle mozzarella and serve.

Nutrition Info: Calories: 393 kcal Fat: 13 g Protein: 13.1 g Carbs: 57.5 g Fiber: 5.9 g

Italian minestrone

Preparation time: 10 minutes

Cooking time: 25 minutes

Servings: 6

Ingredients:

1 tbsp olive oil

1 cup diced celery

1 cup diced yellow onion

1 cup diced carrots

1 cup diced yellow squash

1 cup diced zucchini

1 tbsp minced garlic

2 tbsp tomato paste

4 cups vegetable broth

28 oz diced tomatoes

1 cup dried pasta

1 tsp salt

One bay leaf

Two rosemary sprigs

1 tsp chopped dried oregano

1 cup green beans

15 oz red beans

Black pepper to taste

2 tsp chopped parsley

Directions :

Sauté onions. Carrots and celery in heated olive oil in a Dutch oven over high flame for five minutes. Mix squash and zucchini and cook for two more minutes. Stir in garlic and tomato paste and cook. Pour vegetable stock. Add tomatoes, salt, bay leaf, rosemary, and oregano, and toss well. Let it boil and simmer over medium flame. Mix pasta and red beans and cook for ten minutes. Add greens beans and cook for three minutes. Adjust the consistency of the soup b adding the stock. Adjust the taste and toss well before serving.

Nutrition Info: Calories: 278 kcal Fat: 7 g Protein: 13 g Carbs: 44 g Fiber: 11 g

Asparagus medley

Preparation time: 10 minutes

Cooking time: 30 minutes

Servings: 3

Ingredients:

2 cups cooked pasta

1 cup chopped dill

½ cup chopped cilantro

½ cup chopped mint

4 tbsp olive oil

4 tbsp olive oil

4 tbsp lemon juice

One sliced shallot

Black pepper

1 tbsp cumin

2 cups asparagus

Salt

1.50 cups corn

½ cup chickpeas

1 cup of water

1.5 cups spinach

6 tbsp yogurt

½ tbsp sumac

Directions :

Cook pasta accordingly. Cook shallots, cumin, corn, asparagus, chickpeas, and pepper in heated oil for ten minutes over medium flame. Mix spinach and cook. Add water and simmer it for five minutes. Add pasta and toss well. Transfer the pasta mixture to a bowl and mix mint, cilantro, dill, and drizzle oil.

Nutrition Info: Calories: 317 kcal Fat: 13 g Protein: 9 g Carbs: 43 g Fiber: 6 g

Turmeric Spiced Ginger Cauliflower

Preparation time: 5 minutes

Cook time: 20 minutes

Servings: 4

Ingredients:

One chopped jalapeno

1 tbsp Black mustard seeds

One head cauliflower (cut in florets)

3 tbsp Vegetable oil

1 tbsp grated ginger

1 tsp Turmeric

Salt to taste

Directions :

Mix all the ingredients in a bowl and toss well. Bake in a preheated oven at 425 degrees for 25 minutes.

Nutrition Info: Calories: 139 kcal Fat: 11 g Protein: 3 g Carbs: 9 g Fiber: 5 g

Haystacks

Preparation Time: 10 minutes

Cooking Time: 0 minutes

Serving: 15 cookies

Ingredients:

12 oz. chocolate chips

4 cups chow mien noodle

11 oz. butterscotch chips

Directions :

Melt butterscotch and chips followed by mixing in noodles.

Refrigerator the mixture for 20 minutes and serve.

Nutrition Info: Calories: 267 kcal Fat: 11 g Protein: 2 g Carbs: 38 g Fiber: 0 g

Banana Cheesecake Chocolate Cookies

Preparation Time: 20 Minutes

Cooking Time: 25 Minutes

Serving: 14 cookies

Ingredients:

Crust

2 tbsp butter

12 cookies Oreo

Cheesecakes

1 tsp vanilla extract

2 tbsp flour

1/4 cup cream

1/2 cup sugar

1/2 cup chocolate chips

2 * 8 oz. cream cheese

1/2 cup banana

One egg

Chocolate Whipped Cream

1 cup heavy whipping cream

1/4 cup cocoa powder

2 Tablespoons mini chocolate chips

1/2 cup powdered sugar

1/2 teaspoon rum extract

One yellow banana, sliced

Directions :

Blend all the mixture in the blender except eggs and banana. Now whisk egg and banana and make a batter. Bake the batter in the oven at 350 degrees for twenty-five minutes. Top the cookies with cocoa, cream, vanilla, and sugar mixture. Serve and enjoy.

Nutrition Info: Calories: 351 kcal Fat: 25 g Protein: 4 g Carbs: 31 g Fiber: 0 g

Chocolate Cheesecake Shake

Preparation Time: 10 Minutes

Cooking Time: 0 Minutes

Serving: 4

Ingredients

Six scoops of ice cream (chocolate flavor)

8 oz. cream cheese

2 cups of milk

Directions :

Blend milk and cream cheese in a food processor. Transfer the mixture to a serving glass and add ice cream and serve.

Nutrition Info: Calories: 227 kcal Fat: 16 g Protein: 8 g Carbs: 16 g Fiber: 0 g

Pistachio Milk-Shake

Preparation Time: 5 Minutes

Cooking Time: 0 Minutes

Serving: 4 glasses

Ingredients

1 tsp vanilla extract

4 tbsp pistachios

5 cups ice cream (pistachio)

Pinch of salt

1 cup milk

Directions :

Mix all the ingredients in a blender and serve.

Nutrition Info: Calories: 400 kcal Fat: 26 g Protein: 9 g Carbs: 30 g Fiber: 0 g

Candied Corn Puffs

Preparation Time: 15 Minutes

Cooking Time: 35 Minutes

Serving: 8

Ingredients

8 oz corn puffs

1 cup butter

Salt as required

1 tsp baking soda

1 cup peanuts

1 cup of sugar

1.2 cup of corn syrup

Directions :

Boil syrup, butter, and sugar. Add baking soda and transfer the mixture to a bowl with corn and peanuts. Bake for 35 minutes in the oven at 250 degrees.

Nutrition Info: Calories: 631 kcal Fat: 42 g Protein: 6.2 g Carbs: 62 g Fiber: 0.1 g

Cucumber and Ranch Dressing

Preparation Time: 5 Minutes

Cooking Time: 0 Minutes

Serving: 4

Ingredients

½ chopped onion

¼ tsp pepper and salt each

Two sliced cucumbers

½ tsp dill

½ cup ranch dressing

Directions :

Whisk all the ingredients in a large bowl and set aside.

Serve for 40 minutes.

Nutrition Info: Calories: 232 kcal Fat: 21 g Protein: 2 g Carbs: 12 g Fiber: 0 g

Baked cheese crisp

Preparation Time: 5 Minutes

Cooking Time: 8 Minutes

Serving: 4

Ingredients

¾ cup shredded cheddar

¾ cup parmesan cheese

1 tsp Italian seasoning

Directions :

Mix cheese and place on a baking tray. Bake for eight minutes in the oven at 400 degrees.

Nutrition Info: Calories: 152 kcal Fat: 11 g Protein: 12 g Carbs: 1 g Fiber: 0.2 g

Strawberry Vinaigrette

Preparation Time: 10 minutes

Cooking time: 0 minutes

Servings: 9

Ingredients

8 oz strawberries

Salt to taste

2 tbsp apple cider vinegar

2 tbsp honey

2 tbsp olive oil

¼ tsp black pepper

Directions :

Blend all the ingredients in a blender and pour in the serving dish.

Nutrition Info: Calories: 50 kcal Fat: 3 g Protein: 0.1 g Carbs: 5 g Fiber: 0.8 g

Asian Chicken Salad Wraps

Preparations Time: 20 minutes

Cooking time: 0 minutes

Servings: 6

Ingredients

3 cup cooked chicken breasts-shredded

1/2 cup shredded carrot

¾ tsp minced gingerroot

3 tbsp seasoned rice vinegar

3 tbsp canola oil

2 tbsp honey

1 cup shredded cabbage

1 tbsp water

One chopped garlic clove

¼ tsp pepper

Four chopped green onions

1 cup cilantro leaves

Six lettuce leaves

Six whole-wheat tortillas

Directions :

Whisk all the ingredients in a large mixing bowl and set aside. Place lettuce on each tortilla and spread the chicken mixture, and fold and serve.

Nutrition Info: Calories: 370 kcal Fat: 13 g Protein: 26 g Carbs: 14 g Fiber: 2 g

Buttery Garlic Green Beans

Preparation Time: 10 minutes

Cooking Time: 10 minutes

Servings: 4

Ingredients

1 lb. green beans

Three minced garlic cloves

3 tbsp butter

Lemon pepper to taste

Salt to taste

Directions :

Boil beans in water for seven minutes.

Sauté cooked beans in butter for five minutes over medium flame.

Stir in garlic and cook for five more minutes.

Nutrition Info: Calories: 116 kcal Fat: 8.8 g Protein: 23 g Carbs: 9 g Fiber: 8 g

Hamburger salad

Preparation time: 12 minutes

Cooking time: 10 minutes.

Serving: 4

Ingredients

Sauce

1 tbsp chopped onions

3/4 tbsp vinegar

one cup Mayonnaise

1/2 tsp paprika

2 tsp swerve

2.25 tbsp Dill Pickles

4 tsp Mustard

Salad

1/4 cup dill pickles

1 lb ground beef

kosher salt to taste

4 cups chopped lettuce

Half cup sliced onions

3/4 cup cheddar cheese

black pepper to taste

Directions :

Whisk all the ingredients of the dressing list in a bowl and keep it aside. The dressing is ready.

Cook beef for ten minutes over medium flame in black pepper and salt. Transfer cooked beef in a bowl, add lettuce, pickles, onions, cheese, and toss well. Transfer the dressing to the beef mixture and mix well to coat.

Nutrition Info: Calories: 625 kcal Fat: 52 g Protein: 31 g Carbs: 5 g Fiber: 3 g

Pork tacos

Preparation time: 10 minutes

Cooking time: 20 minutes

Serving: 6

Ingredients

1 tsp toasted cumin

1.5 lb sliced pork

Salt to taste 1.75 tsp ground guajillo

3 tbsp olive oil

Black pepper to taste

Three minced garlic cloves

Serving

24 tortillas

Salsa cruda

As needed, Cilantro sprigs

Tomatillo salsa

Radishes

Directions :

Sprinkle spices over pork pieces to marinate it.

Cook pork in heated oil over medium flame for ten minutes.

Place them aside.

Toast tortillas in skillet. Now, place cooked pork, tomatillo salsa, radish, cruda salsa, and cilantro and serve.

Nutrition Info: Calories: 330 kcal Fat: 27 g Protein: 20 g Carbs: 1 g Fiber: 18 g

Broccoli blossom

Preparation time: 5 minutes

Cooking time: 15 minutes

Servings: 2

Ingredients

tbsp oil

One chopped cabbage

¼ cup chopped onion

½ cup sliced broccoli

¼ tsp tarragon tbsp water

¼ tsp garlic and onion powder

Red pepper to taste

Black pepper as required

One toasted muffin tbsp cheese

Directions :

Heat oil in a skillet and sauté veggies for five minutes.

Pour in water and simmer for six minutes. Add all the spices and

toss well. Spread the sauce over muffins and drizzle cheese

before serving.

Nutrition Info: Calories: 297 kcal Fat: 16 g Protein: 24 g

Carbs: 20 g Fiber: 8 g

Spicy Kenyan greens

Preparation time: 10 minutes

Cooking time: 15 minutes

Servings: 6

Ingredients

One cup of water

One jalapeno pepper

Salt to taste

2 tbsp black pepper

2 tbsp olive oil lb chopped collards

10 oz chopped turnip tbsp butter

Three chopped tomatoes

One chopped onion

7 oz milk tsp roasted peanuts

Directions :

Combine olive oil, salt, water, chili pepper in a pot and cook over medium heat.

Add greens to the boiling mixture for five minutes. Drain and place aside. Melt butter in a skillet and sauté cooked greens, tomatoes, milk, and onions in it for five minutes. Sprinkle salt, pepper, and peanuts and serve.

Nutrition Info: Calories: 284 kcal Fat: 26 g Protein: 6 g Carbs: 12 g Fiber: 6 g

Coconut curry cauliflower

Preparation time: 5 minutes

Cooking time: 25 minutes

Servings: 4

Ingredients

2 tbsp olive oil

½ chopped cauliflower

¼ tsp salt tsp curry paste coconut milk

¼ cup chopped cilantro

1 tbsp lime juice

Directions :

Sauté cauliflower in heated olive oil over medium flame for ten minutes.

Mix milk and curry powder and simmer for ten minutes.

Add lime juice and cilantro and toss well.

Serve and enjoy it.

Nutrition Info: Calories: 243 kcal Fat: 24 g Protein: 3 g Carbs: 9 g Fiber: 2 g

Sicilian Spaghetti

Preparation time: 10 minutes

Cooking time: 5 minutes

Servings: 8

Ingredients

4 tbsp cheese

One lb spaghetti

Three minced garlic cloves

4 tbsp olive oil

2 oz anchovy fillets

One cup parsley

One cup bread crumbs

Black pepper to taste

Directions :

Cook pasta for ten minutes in boiling water over medium flame in a large deep pot.

Cook anchovies and garlic in heated olive oil for three minutes with constant stirring. Mix breadcrumbs, pepper, and parsley in the mixture. Mix anchovy with the pasta and spread cheese before serving.

108

Nutrition Info: : Calories: 354 kcal Fat: 10 g Protein: 13 g Carbs: 53.6 g Fiber: 3 g

www.ingramcontent.com/pod-product-compliance
Lightning Source LLC
Chambersburg PA
CBHW061003050726
47592CB00003B/1319